99 Headache and Migraine Juice and Meal Recipe Solutions:

Reduce Pain Fast and Permanently

By

Joe Correa CSN

COPYRIGHT

This publication is designed to provide accurate and authoritative information in regard to the subject matter covered. It is sold with the understanding that neither the author nor the publisher is engaged in rendering medical advice. If medical advice or assistance is needed, consult with a doctor. This book is considered a guide and should not be used in any way detrimental to your health. Consult with a physician before starting this nutritional plan to make sure it's right for you.

ACKNOWLEDGEMENTS

This book is dedicated to my friends and family that have had mild or serious illnesses so that you may find a solution and make the necessary changes in your life.

99 Headache and Migraine Juice and Meal Recipe Solutions:

Reduce Pain Fast and Permanently

By

Joe Correa CSN

CONTENTS

ABOUT THE AUTHOR

After years of Research, I honestly believe in the positive effects that proper nutrition can have over the body and mind. My knowledge and experience has helped me live healthier throughout the years and which I have shared with family and friends. The more you know about eating and drinking healthier, the sooner you will want to change your life and eating habits.

Nutrition is a key part in the process of being healthy and living longer so get started today. The first step is the most important and the most significant.

INTRODUCTION

99 Headache and Migraine Juice and Meal Recipe Solutions: Reduce Pain Fast and Permanently

By Joe Correa CSN

I have learned that every individual has his or her own triggers that cause headaches. Some people have bad reactions to certain dairy products, eggs, meat, chocolate, etc., without them being aware that these foods can increase the amount of headaches they will have. However, salmon is known as an omega 3 fatty acid booster, and it's proven to help with inflammation which leads to migraines and headaches.

You should experiment with the food you eat and learn to listen to what your body has to tell you. For example, if you eat large amounts of a certain food and your headache appears, then you should remove it from your diet.

Headaches are a common problem people experience all the time during their life. Usually, they appear and disappear spontaneously not causing any serious problems or damage. In these cases, headaches are related to stress, problems with blood vessels, nervous system, physical inactivity, or problems with the muscles of the neck or eyes.

Knowing the difference between a headache and a migraine is extremely important because it can mean a better treatment method and prevent future pain from occurring in the first place.

Unlike traditional, low-intensity headaches that come and go without any pattern, migraines are more painful and is often a more severe type of headache. It's followed by some standard symptoms that include nausea, vomiting, sensitivity to light behind one eye or ear, and even temporary vision loss. In some cases, people experience such severe headaches that they are hospitalized.

As someone who has been able to eliminate chronic headaches, I have found that eating plenty of fresh fruits and vegetables every single day helped me put things under control. Also, increase water consumption and reduce red meat consumption.

This book offers a collection of juice and meal recipes that will help you deal with this problem. Meat is minimized in the recipes because it contributes to a hormonal imbalance which is one of the most significant triggers for headaches and migraines. Try them all and see which ones help you to reduce headaches and migraines the fastest.

99 HEADACHE AND MIGRAINE JUICE AND MEAL RECIPE SOLUTIONS: REDUCE PAIN FAST AND PERMANENTLY

JUICES

1.   Apple Kiwi Juice

Ingredients:

1 Red Delicious apple, cored and chopped

1 whole kiwi, peeled and chopped

1 cup of blueberries

1 whole lemon, halved

¼ tsp of ginger, ground

1 oz of water

Preparation:

Wash the apple and cut lengthwise in half. Remove the core and cut into bite-sized pieces and set aside.

Peel the kiwi and cut into small pieces. Make sure to reserve the kiwi juice while cutting.

Place the blueberries in a colander. Rinse well under cold running water and drain. Fill the measuring cup and reserve the rest in the refrigerator.

Peel the lemon and cut lengthwise in half. Set aside.

Now, combine apple, kiwi, blueberries, and lemon in a juicer and process until juiced. Transfer to a serving glass and stir in the ginger, water, and reserved kiwi juice.

Add some crushed ice and serve immediately.

Nutrition information per serving: Kcal: 217, Protein: 3.2g, Carbs: 66.2g, Fats: 1.3g

2.   Green Coconut Juice

Ingredients:

1 cup of beet greens, torn

1 cup of kale, chopped

1 cup of parsley, chopped

2 small cucumbers, peeled

1 whole lime, peeled and halved

1 tbsp of agave syrup

3 tbsp of coconut water

Preparation:

Combine beet greens, kale, and parsley in a large colander. Rinse under cold running water and drain. Chop into small pieces and set aside.

Wash the cucumber and cut into thin slices. Set aside.

Peel the lime and cut lengthwise in half. Set aside.

Now, combine beet greens, kale, parsley, cucumber, and lime in a juicer. Process until juiced. Transfer to a serving glass and stir in the agave and coconut water.

Mix well and serve cold.

Nutrition information per serving: Kcal: 139, Protein: 10.6g, Carbs: 42.2g, Fats: 1.9g

3. Pear Raspberry Juice

Ingredients:

3 large pears, cored and chopped

1 cup of fresh raspberries

1 medium-sized beet, trimmed

1 large lemon, peeled

1 oz of water

Preparation:

Wash the pear and cut in half. Remove the core and cut into bite-sized pieces. Set aside.

Rinse the raspberries in a colander and drain. Set aside.

Wash the beet and trim off the green parts. Peel and chop into bite-sized pieces. Set aside.

Peel the lemon and cut lengthwise in half. Set aside.

Now, combine pear, raspberries, beet, and lemon in a juicer. Process until juiced.

Transfer to a serving glass and stir in the water. Add some crushed ice and serve immediately.

Nutrition information per serving: Kcal: 378, Protein: 2.7g, Carbs: 133g, Fats: 2.7g

4.   Swiss Chard Apple Juice

Ingredients:

1 cup of Swiss chard, chopped

1 large green apple, cored

1 cup of fresh basil, chopped

1 large lemon, peeled

1 cup of fresh mint, chopped

2 oz of water

Preparation:

Combine basil, Swiss chard, and mint in a large colander. Wash thoroughly under cold running water. Chop into small pieces and set aside.

Wash the apple and cut in half. Remove the core and cut into bite-sized pieces. Set aside.

Peel the lemon and cut lengthwise in half.

Now, combine Swiss chard, apple, basil, mint, and lemon in a juicer and process until well juiced. Transfer to serving glasses and stir in the water.

Refrigerate for 5 minutes before serving.

Enjoy!

Nutrition information per serving: Kcal: 126, Protein: 3.9g, Carbs: 39.1g, Fats: 1.1g

5.   Carrot Watercress Juice

Ingredients:

2 large carrots, sliced

1 cup of watercress, torn

1 cup of pineapple, chunked

1 large lime, peeled

1 small ginger knob, peeled

2 oz of water

Preparation:

Wash and peel the carrots. Cut into thin slices and set aside.

Wash the watercress thoroughly under cold running water. Torn with hands and set aside.

Cut the top of a pineapple and peel it with sharp cutting knife. Chop into small chunks and set aside.

Peel the lime and cut lengthwise in half. Set aside.

Peel the ginger root knob and cut into small pieces. Set aside.

Now, combine carrots, watercress, pineapple, lemon, and ginger in a juicer and process until well juiced.

Transfer to serving glasses and stir in water.

Add some ice and serve.

Nutrition information per serving: Kcal: 135, Protein: 3.3g, Carbs: 40.6g, Fats: 3.3g

6.   Celery Turmeric Juice

Ingredients:

1 cup of celery, chopped

¼ tsp of turmeric, ground

1 cup of asparagus, trimmed

1 large green bell pepper, chopped

¼ tsp of ginger, ground

1 oz of water

Preparation:

Wash the celery and chop into small pieces. Set aside.

Wash the asparagus and trim off the woody ends. Cut into small pieces and fill the measuring cup. Reserve the rest in the refrigerator.

Wash the bell pepper and cut lengthwise in half. Remove the stem and seeds. Chop into small pieces and set aside.

Now, combine celery, asparagus, pepper, in a juicer and process until well juiced. Transfer to a serving glass and stir in the turmeric, ginger, and water.

Add some ice and serve immediately.

Enjoy!

Nutrition information per serving: Kcal: 48, Protein: 5.1g, Carbs: 15.8g, Fats: 0.6g

7.   Apple Asparagus Juice

Ingredients:

1 large Granny Smith's apple, cored

1 cup of fresh asparagus, trimmed

3 medium-sized oranges, peeled and wedged

¼ tsp of turmeric, ground

2 oz of water

Preparation:

Peel the oranges and divide into wedges. Set aside.

Wash the apple and remove the core. Cut into bite-sized pieces and set aside.

Wash the asparagus thoroughly under cold running water and trim off the woody ends. Cut into small pieces and set aside.

Now, combine apple, asparagus, and oranges in a juicer and process until juiced. Transfer to serving glasses and stir in the turmeric and water.

Refrigerate for 5 minutes before serving.

Nutrition information per serving: Kcal: 316, Protein: 9.1g, Carbs: 98.1g, Fats: 1.2g

8.   Pear Pepper Juice

Ingredients:

1 large pear, cored and chopped

1 large red bell pepper, chopped

2 cups of beets, chopped

1 large lemon, peeled

1 small ginger root slice, peeled

2 oz of water

Preparation:

Wash the pear and cut in half. Remove the core and cut into bite-sized pieces. Set aside.

Wash the bell pepper and cut in half. Remove the seeds and cut into small pieces. Set aside.

Wash the beets and trim off the green ends. Cut into small pieces and fill the measuring cup. Reserve the greens for some other juice. Set aside.

Peel the lemon and cut lengthwise in half. Set aside.

Peel the ginger slice and cut in half. Set aside.

Now, combine pear, bell pepper, beets, lemon, and ginger in a juicer. Process until well juiced and transfer to serving glasses.

Stir in the water and add some ice before serving.

Enjoy!

Nutrition information per serving: Kcal: 239, Protein: 7.5g, Carbs: 76.7g, Fats: 1.4g

9.   Avocado Kale Juice

Ingredients:

1 cup of avocado, cubed

1 cup of fresh kale, torn

2 cups of Iceberg lettuce, torn

1 whole kiwi, peeled and halved

1 whole cucumber, sliced

Preparation:

Peel the avocado and cut lengthwise in half. Remove the pit and cut into small cubes. Fill the measuring cup and reserve the rest for later.

Combine kale and lettuce in a large colander. Wash thoroughly under cold running water and torn into small pieces. Set aside.

Peel the kiwi and cut lengthwise in half. Set aside.

Wash the cucumber and cut into thin slices. Fill the measuring cup and reserve the rest for later.

Now, combine avocado, kale, lettuce, kiwi, and cucumber in a juicer and process until juiced. Transfer to a serving glass and add some ice before serving.

Enjoy!

Nutrition information per serving: Kcal: 304, Protein: 9.8g, Carbs: 42.8g, Fats: 23.6g

10.   Spinach Watercress Juice

Ingredients:

2 cups of spinach, torn

1 cup of watercress, torn

1 cup of kale, torn

1 cup of Swiss chard, torn

¼ tsp of ginger, ground

1 oz of water

Preparation:

Combine, spinach, watercress, kale, and Swiss chard in a large colander. Wash thoroughly under cold running water. Slightly drain and torn into small pieces.

Now, transfer the greens to a juicer and process until juiced. Transfer to a serving glass and stir in the ginger and water.

Refrigerate for 10 minutes before serving.

Enjoy!

Nutrition information per serving: Kcal: 87, Protein: 16.3g, Carbs: 22.9g, Fats: 2.4g

11.   Banana Apple Juice

Ingredients:

1 cup of pomegranate seeds

1 large banana, chopped

1 small Granny Smith's apple, cored

1 cup of raspberries

¼ tsp of ginger, ground

Preparation:

Peel the banana and cut into small pieces. Set aside.

Wash the apple and cut lengthwise in half. Remove the core and cut into bite-sized pieces. Set aside.

Cut the top of the pomegranate fruit using a sharp paring knife. Slice down to each of the white membranes inside of the fruit. Pop the seeds into a measuring cup and set aside.

Rinse the raspberries under cold running water using a colander. Drain and set aside.

Now, combine banana, apple, pomegranate seeds, and raspberries in a juicer and process until juiced. Transfer to a serving glass and stir in the ginger.

Add some ice and serve immediately.

Nutrition information per serving: Kcal: 265, Protein: 5.1g, Carbs: 81.6g, Fats: 2.5g

12.   Blackberry Mint Juice

Ingredients:

1 cup of blackberries

1 cup of fresh mint, chopped

1 whole lime, peeled

1 cup of pineapple, chunked

2 oz of coconut water

Preparation:

Place the blackberries in a large colander. Rinse thoroughly under cold running water. Drain and set aside.

Wash the mint and drain. Chop into small pieces and set aside.

Peel the lime and cut lengthwise in half. Set aside.

Using a sharp paring knife, cut the top of the pineapple. Gently remove all hard skin and slice it into thin slices. Fill the measuring cup and reserve the rest for later.

Now, combine blackberries, mint, lime, and pineapple in a juicer. Process until well juiced and transfer to a serving glass.

Stir in the coconut water and add few ice cubes before serving. Enjoy!

Nutrition information per serving: Kcal: 125, Protein: 4g, Carbs: 42.9g, Fats: 1.2g

13.   Orange Grape Juice

Ingredients:

1 large red orange, peeled

1 cup of green grapes

1 cup of beets, trimmed and sliced

1 whole apricot, pitted

1 tbsp of coconut water

Preparation:

Peel the orange and divide into wedges. Cut each wedge in half and set aside.

Rinse the grapes and remove the stems. Set aside.

Wash the beets and trim off the green parts. Cut into thin slices and fill the measuring cup. Reserve the rest for later.

Wash the apricot and cut lengthwise in half. Remove the pit and cut into small pieces. Set aside.

Now, combine orange, grapes, beets, and apricots in a juicer and process until well juiced. Transfer to a serving glass and stir in the coconut water.

Add some ice and serve immediately.

Nutrition information per serving: Kcal: 184, Protein: 4.9g, Carbs: 54.3g, Fats: 0.9g

14. Lemon Watermelon Juice

Ingredients:

1 whole lemon, peeled

1 cup of watermelon, chunked

1 large pear, chopped

1 cup of cranberries

¼ tsp of cinnamon, ground

1 oz of water

Preparation:

Peel the lemon and cut lengthwise in half. Set aside.

Cut the watermelon in half. Cut one large wedge and wrap the rest in a plastic foil and refrigerate. Peel the slice and cut into small cubes. Remove the pits and fill the measuring cup. Set aside.

Wash the pear and cut in half. Remove the core and cut into small pieces. Set aside.

Place the cranberries in a colander and rinse under cold running water. Drain and set aside.

Now, combine lemon, watermelon, pear, and cranberries

in a juicer and process until well juiced. Transfer to a serving glass and stir in the cinnamon and water.

Refrigerate for 5 minutes before serving.

Nutrition information per serving: Kcal: 186, Protein: 2.8g, Carbs: 64.1g, Fats: 0.8g

15.   Plum Cantaloupe Juice

Ingredients:

1 whole plum, chopped

1 cup of cantaloupe, chopped

1 large orange, peeled

1 cup of fresh mint, torn

¼ tsp of ginger, ground

Preparation:

Wash the plum and cut in half. Remove the pit and chop into small pieces. Set aside.

Cut the cantaloupe in half. Scoop out the seeds and flesh. Cut and peel one large wedge. Chop into chunks and fill the measuring cup. Reserve the rest of the cantaloupe in a refrigerator.

Peel the orange and divide into wedges. Cut each wedge in half and set aside.

Wash the mint thoroughly under cold running water. Torn into small pieces and set aside.

Now, combine orange, plum, cantaloupe, and mint in a

juicer and process until juiced. Transfer to a serving glass and stir in the ginger.

Add some ice and serve immediately.

Enjoy!

Nutrition information per serving: Kcal: 151, Protein: 4.4g, Carbs: 45.6g, Fats: 0.9g

16.   Banana Lime Juice

Ingredients:

1 large banana, chopped

1 whole lime, peeled

1 cup of watermelon, chopped

1 cup of fresh mint, torn

1 small Granny Smith's apple, cored

¼ tsp of cinnamon, ground

Preparation:

Peel the banana and cut into small chunks. Set aside.

Peel the lime and cut lengthwise in half. Set aside.

Cut the watermelon in half. Cut one large wedge and wrap the rest in a plastic foil and refrigerate. Peel the slice and cut into small cubes. Remove the pits and fill the measuring cup. Set aside.

Wash the mint thoroughly under cold running water. Drain and torn into small pieces. Set aside.

Wash the apple and cut lengthwise in half. Remove the core and chop into bite-sized pieces. Set aside.

Now, combine banana, lime, watermelon, mint, and apple in a juicer and process until juiced. Transfer to a serving glass and stir in the cinnamon.

Add some crushed Ice and serve immediately.

Nutrition information per serving: Kcal: 239, Protein: 4.2g, Carbs: 69.5g, Fats: 1.2g

17.   Blackberry Apple Juice

Ingredients:

1 cup of blackberries

1 small Golden Delicious apple, cored

1 cup of strawberries, chopped

1 large pear, chopped

¼ tsp of cinnamon, ground

1 oz of water

Preparation:

Wash the blackberries using a colander. Drain and set aside.

Wash the apple and cut lengthwise in half. Remove the core and chop into bite-sized pieces. Set aside.

Wash the strawberries and remove the stems. Cut into small pieces and fill the measuring cup. Reserve the rest in the refrigerator.

Wash the pear and cut in half. Remove the core and cut into small pieces. Set aside.

Now, combine blackberries, apple, strawberries, and pear

in a juicer and process until well juiced. Transfer to a serving glass and stir in the cinnamon.

Refrigerate for 5 minutes before serving.

Enjoy!

Nutrition information per serving: Kcal: 246, Protein: 4.2g, Carbs: 82.1g, Fats: 1.7g

18. Fennel Apple Juice

Ingredients:

1 cup of fennel, chopped

1 small Granny Smith's apple, cored

1 large orange, peeled

1 cup of blueberries

¼ tsp of ginger, ground

Preparation:

Trim off the outer wilted layers of the fennel. Roughly chop it and fill the measuring cup. Reserve the rest for later.

Wash the apple and cut lengthwise in half. Remove the core and cut into bite-sized pieces. Set aside.

Peel the orange and divide into wedges. Cut each wedge in half and set aside.

Place the blueberries in a colander and wash thoroughly under cold running water. Drain and set aside.

Now, combine fennel, apple, orange, and blueberries in a juicer and process until juiced. Transfer to a serving glass and stir in the ginger.

Add few ice cubes and serve immediately.

Enjoy!

Nutrition information per serving: Kcal: 222, Protein: 4.5g, Carbs: 69.1g, Fats: 1.5g

19.   Spinach Pomegranate Juice

Ingredients:

1 cup of fresh spinach, torn

1 cup of pomegranate seeds

1 cup of sweet potato, cubed

1 whole lemon, peeled

2 oz of water

Preparation:

Wash the spinach thoroughly under cold running water. Drain and torn into small pieces. Set aside.

Cut the top of the pomegranate fruit using a sharp paring knife. Slice down to each of the white membranes inside of the fruit. Pop the seeds into a measuring cup and set aside.

Peel the sweet potato and cut into small cubes. Place in a deep pot and add 3 cups of water. Bring it to a boil and cook for 5 minutes. Remove from the heat and drain. Set aside.

Peel the lemon and cut lengthwise in half. Set aside.

Now, combine spinach, pomegranate seeds, previously cooked potato, and lemon in a juicer. Process until well juiced.

Transfer to a serving glass and stir in the water. Add some ice and serve immediately.

Enjoy!

Nutrition information per serving: Kcal: 195, Protein: 10.2g, Carbs: 56.1g, Fats: 2.1g

20. Watermelon Banana Juice

Ingredients:

1 large wedge of watermelon

1 large banana, sliced

1 cup of strawberries, chopped

2 whole plums, pitted

Preparation:

Cut the watermelon in half. Cut one large wedge and wrap the rest in a plastic foil and refrigerate. Peel the slice and cut into small cubes. Remove the pits and fill the measuring cup. Set aside.

Peel the banana and cut into thin slices. Set aside.

Wash the strawberries and remove the stems. Cut into small pieces and fill the measuring cup. Reserve the rest for in the refrigerator.

Wash the plums and cut into halves. Remove the pits and cut into small pieces. Set aside.

Now, combine watermelon, banana, strawberries, and plums in a juicer and process until juiced. Transfer to a serving glass and add some ice.

Serve immediately.

Nutrition information per serving: Kcal: 273, Protein: 5.1g, Carbs: 78.8g, Fats: 1.6g

21.   Asparagus Collard Green Juice

Ingredients:

1 cup of asparagus, trimmed and chopped

1 cup of collard greens, torn

1 medium-sized tomato, chopped

1 cup of spinach, torn

¼ tsp salt

1 rosemary sprig

Preparation:

Wash the asparagus and trim off the woody ends. Cut into small pieces and fill the measuring cup. Set aside.

Combine collard greens and spinach in a large colander. Wash under cold running water and drain. Torn into small pieces and set aside.

Wash the tomato and place it in a small bowl. Cut into small pieces and reserve the tomato juice while cutting. Set aside.

Now, combine asparagus, collard greens, tomato, and spinach in a juicer and process until juiced. Transfer to a serving glass and stir in the reserve tomato juice and salt. Sprinkle with rosemary.

Serve immediately.

Nutrition information per serving: Kcal: 66, Protein: 11.2g, Carbs: 19.6g, Fats: 1.5g

22.   Strawberry Apple Juice

Ingredients:

1 cup of strawberries, chopped

1 small Granny Smith's apple, cored and chopped

1 whole guava, chunked

1 whole lemon, peeled and halved

¼ tsp of cinnamon, ground

2 oz of water

Preparation:

Wash the strawberries and remove the stems. Cut into small pieces and fill the measuring cup. Reserve the rest in the refrigerator. Set aside.

Wash the apple and cut lengthwise in half. Remove the core and cut into bite-sized pieces. Set aside.

Peel the guava and cut in half. Scoop out the seeds and wash it. Cut into small chunks and set aside.

Peel the lemon and cut lengthwise in half. Set aside.

Now, combine strawberries, apple, guava, and lemon in a juicer and process until juiced. Transfer to a serving glass and stir in the cinnamon and water.

Refrigerate for 10 minutes before serving.

Enjoy!

Nutrition information per serving: Kcal: 136, Protein: 3.6g, Carbs: 43.9g, Fats: 1.3g

23.   Lettuce Cabbage Juice

Ingredients:

1 cup of red leaf lettuce, chopped

1 cup of purple cabbage, chopped

1 medium-sized artichoke, chopped

1 cup of fresh basil, torn

1 cup of cucumber, sliced

1 large carrot, sliced

Preparation:

Combine lettuce and cabbage in a large colander and rinse well under cold running water. Drain and chop into small pieces. Set aside.

Trim off the outer layers of the artichoke using a sharp paring knife. Cut into bite-sized pieces and set aside.

Rinse the basil with cold water and torn into small pieces. Set aside.

Wash the cucumber and cut into thin slices. Fill the measuring cup and reserve the rest in the refrigerator.

Wash and peel the carrot. Cut into thin slices and set aside.

Now, combine lettuce, cabbage, artichoke, basil, cucumber, and carrot in a juicer and process until juiced.

Transfer to a serving glass and serve immediately.

Nutrition information per serving: Kcal: 88, Protein: 7.6g, Carbs: 30.1g, Fats: 0.7g

24.   Cherry Banana Juice

Ingredients:

1 cup of cherries, pitted

1 large banana, peeled

1 cup of blueberries

1 whole lemon, peeled

1 small Granny Smith's apple, cored

¼ tsp of cinnamon

Preparation:

Wash the cherries and cut in half. Remove the pits and stems. Set aside.

Peel the banana and cut into small chunks. Set aside.

Rinse the blueberries using a large colander. Drain and set aside.

Peel the lemon and cut lengthwise in half. Set aside.

Wash the apple and cut lengthwise in half. Remove the core and cut into small pieces. Set aside.

Now, combine cherries, banana, blueberries, lemon, and

apple in a juicer and process until juiced. Transfer to a serving glass and stir in the cinnamon.

Add some ice and serve immediately.

Nutrition information per serving: Kcal: 340, Protein: 5.5g, Carbs: 102g, Fats: 1.7g

25.   Banana Celery Juice

Ingredients:

1 medium-sized banana, sliced

1 medium-sized celery stalk, chopped

3 whole apricots, chopped

1 small apple, chopped

Preparation:

Peel the banana and cut into small chunks. Set aside.

Wash the celery stalk and cut into bite-sized pieces. Set aside.

Wash the apricots and cut in half. Remove the pits and cut into bite-sized pieces. Set aside.

Wash the apple and cut in half. Remove the core and cut into bite-sized pieces. Set aside.

Now, combine banana, celery, apricots, and apple in a juicer and process until juiced. Transfer to a serving glass and add some ice.

Serve immediately.

Nutrition information per serving: Kcal: 154, Protein: 3.5g, Carbs: 45.8g, Fats: 1.1g

26. Cucumber Onion Juice

Ingredients:

1 cup of cucumber, chopped

1 spring onion, chopped

1 medium-sized tomato, chopped

1 yellow bell pepper, chopped

¼ tsp of Himalayan salt

3 oz of water

Preparation:

Place the tomato in a bowl and cut into quarters. Reserve the tomato juice while cutting and set aside.

Wash the bell pepper and cut in half. Remove the seeds and cut into small pieces. Set aside.

Wash the cucumber and cut into thick slices.

Wash the spring onion and chop it into small pieces. Set aside.

Now, combine cucumber, onion, tomato, and bell pepper in a juicer and process until juiced.

Transfer to a serving glasses and stir in the salt, water, and reserved tomato juice.

Add some ice cubes before serving and enjoy!

Nutrition information per serving: Kcal: 73, Protein: 3.7g, Carbs: 20.1g, Fats: 0.9g

27.   Zucchini Leek Juice

Ingredients:

1 medium-sized zucchini, peeled

1 whole leek, chopped

1 large green apple, peeled and seeds removed

1 cups of mustard greens, chopped

1 cup of Brussels sprouts

1 cup of parsnip, sliced

¼ tsp of ginger, ground

Preparation:

Wash the zucchini and cut in half. Scoop out the seeds using a spoon. Cut into small chunks and set aside.

Wash the leek and cut into small pieces. Set aside.

Wash the apple and remove the core. Cut into bite-sized pieces and set aside.

Wash the mustard greens and torn with hands. Set aside.

Wash the Brussels sprouts and trim off the outer leaves. Set aside.

Wash the parsnips and cut into thick slices. Set aside.

Now, process zucchini, leek, apple, mustard greens, Brussels sprouts, and parsnips in a juicer.

Transfer to serving glasses and refrigerate for 10 minutes before serving.

Nutrition information per serving: Kcal: 284, Protein: 12.3g, Carbs: 83.7g, Fats: 2.4g

28.   Celery Beet Juice

Ingredients:

1 cup of celery, chopped

1 cup of beets, sliced

1 cup of pomegranate seeds

1 cup of crookneck squash, sliced

1 tbsp of honey

¼ tsp of ginger, ground

Preparation:

Wash the celery and cut into small pieces. Set aside.

Wash the beets and trim off the green parts. Cut into bite-sized pieces and set aside.

Cut the top of the pomegranate fruit using a sharp knife. Slice down to each of the white membranes inside of the fruit. Pop the seeds into a measuring cup and set aside.

Wash the crookneck squash and cut in half. Scoop out the seeds using a spoon. Cut into small chunks and set aside. Reserve the rest for another juice.

Now, process celery, beets, beet greens, pomegranate

seeds, and squash in a juicer.

Transfer to serving glasses and stir in the honey.

Add some ice and serve immediately.

Nutrition information per serving: Kcal: 132, Protein: 6.4g, Carbs: 48.8g, Fats: 1.8g

29.   Orange Carrot Juice

Ingredients:

1 large orange, peeled and wedged

1 large carrot, sliced

1 cup of pumpkin, cubed

1 cup of cucumber, sliced

1 small ginger knob, chopped

Preparation:

Peel the orange and divide into wedges. Cut each wedge in half and set aside.

Wash and peel the carrot. Cut into thin slices and set aside.

Cut the top of a pumpkin. Cut lengthwise in half and then scrape out the seeds. Cut one large wedge and peel it. Cut into small cubes and fill the measuring cup. Reserve the rest in the refrigerator.

Wash the cucumber and cut into thin slices. Fill the measuring cup and reserve the rest for later. Set aside.

Peel the ginger knob and cut into small pieces. Set aside.

Now, combine, orange, carrot, pumpkin, cucumber, and

ginger in a juicer. Process until well juiced. Transfer to a serving glass and add some ice.

Serve immediately.

Nutrition information per serving: Kcal: 130, Protein: 4.1g, Carbs: 39.1g, Fats: 0.6g

30.   Blueberry Lettuce Juice

Ingredients:

1 cup of blueberries

1 cup of Romaine lettuce, shredded

1 whole lime, peeled

1 large banana, sliced

1 whole cucumber, sliced

1 oz of water

Preparation:

Rinse the blueberries using a small colander. Slightly drain and fill the measuring cup. Set aside.

Rinse the lettuce thoroughly under cold running water. Shred it and fill the measuring cup. Set aside.

Peel the lime and cut lengthwise in half. Set aside.

Peel the banana and cut into thin slices. Set aside.

Wash the cucumber and cut into thin slices. Set aside.

Now, combine blueberries, lettuce, lime, banana, and cucumber in a juicer and process until juiced. Transfer to a serving glass and stir in the water. Add some crushed ice and serve immediately.

Nutrition information per serving: Kcal: 176, Protein: 9.8g, Carbs: 49.5g, Fats: 1.7g

31.   Basil Avocado Juice

Ingredients:

1 cup of fresh basil, torn

1 cup of avocado, cut into bite-sized pieces

1 cup of cucumber, sliced

1 medium-sized zucchini, chopped

1 cup of red leaf lettuce, torn

Preparation:

Combine basil and lettuce in a large colander and rinse under cold running water. Drain and torn with hands into small pieces. Set aside.

Peel the avocado and cut lengthwise in half. Remove the pit and cut into bite-sized pieces. Fill the measuring cup and reserve the rest in the refrigerator.

Wash the cucumber and cut into thin slices. Fill the measuring cup and refrigerate for later.

Peel the zucchini and chop into small pieces. Set aside.

Now, combine basil, avocado, cucumber, lettuce, and zucchini in a juicer. Process until well juiced. Transfer to a serving glass and add some ice.

Serve immediately.

Nutrition information per serving: Kcal: 234, Protein: 6.7g, Carbs: 21.7g, Fats: 22.3g

32.   Honey Lemon Juice

Ingredients:

1 tbsp honey, raw

1 whole lemon, peeled

1 cup of strawberries, chopped

1 cup of spinach, torn

1 whole lime, peeled

2 oz of water

Preparation:

Peel the lemon and lime. Cut each fruit lengthwise in half and set aside.

Wash the strawberries and remove the stems. Cut into bite-sized pieces and set aside.

Wash the spinach thoroughly under cold running water. Slightly drain and torn into small pieces. Set aside.

Now, combine spinach, lemon, lime, and strawberries in a juicer and process until juiced. Transfer to a serving glass and stir in the water and honey.

Refrigerate for 5 minutes before serving.

Enjoy!

Nutrition information per serving: Kcal: 81, Protein: 5.8g, Carbs: 27.8g, Fats: 1.4g

33. Cantaloupe Cucumber Juice

Ingredients:

1 cup of cantaloupe, diced

1 medium-sized cucumber, peeled

1 cup of baby spinach, torn

1 cup of cranberries

1 cup of parsley, chopped

1 tbsp of honey, raw

Preparation:

Cut the cantaloupe in half. Scoop out the seeds and flesh. Cut two wedges and peel them. Chop into chunks and set aside. Reserve the rest of the cantaloupe in a refrigerator.

Wash the cucumber and cut into thick slices. Set aside.

Combine spinach and parsley in a colander and wash under cold running water. Torn with hands and set aside.

Wash the cranberries and set aside.

Now, process cantaloupe, cucumber, parsley, baby spinach, and cranberries in a juicer.

Transfer to serving glasses and stir in the honey.

Refrigerate for 5 minutes before serving.

Enjoy!

Nutrition information per serving: Kcal: 197, Protein: 10.2g, Carbs: 58.3g, Fats: 2.2g

34.   Cinnamon Peach Juice

Ingredients:

¼ tsp of cinnamon, ground

1 large peach, pitted and chopped

1 small green apple, cored and chopped

1 whole banana, sliced

1 oz of coconut water

1 tbsp of mint, finely chopped

Preparation:

Wash the peach and cut lengthwise in half. Remove the pit and cut into bite-sized pieces. Set side.

Wash the apple and cut in half. Remove the core and chop into small pieces. Set aside.

Peel the banana and cut into thin slices. Set aside.

Now, combine peach, apple, and bananas in a juicer and process until well juiced. Transfer to a serving glass and stir in the cinnamon and coconut water.

Sprinkle with mint and add ice.

Enjoy!

Nutrition information per serving: Kcal: 362, Protein: 5.5g, Carbs: 104g, Fats: 1.7g

35.   Avocado Ginger Juice

Ingredients:

1 cup of avocado, chopped

1 small ginger knob

1 cup of beets, trimmed

1 large carrot, sliced

¼ tsp turmeric, ground

2 oz water

Preparation:

Peel the avocado and cut lengthwise in half. Remove the pit and cut into bite-sized pieces. Fill the measuring cup and reserve the rest in the refrigerator.

Peel the ginger knob and cut into small pieces. Set aside.

Trim off the green parts of the beets. Slightly peel and cut into thin slices. Fill the measuring cup and refrigerate the rest.

Wash and peel the carrot. Cut into bite-sized pieces and set aside.

Now, combine avocado, ginger, beets, and carrot in a

juicer. Process until well juiced and transfer to a serving glass. Stir in the turmeric and water and refrigerate for 5 minutes before serving.

Enjoy!

Nutrition information per serving: Kcal: 265, Protein: 5.9g, Carbs: 33.4g, Fats: 21.8g

36.   Asparagus Cucumber Juice

Ingredients:

1 cup of asparagus, chopped

1 cup of cucumber, sliced

1 cup of cauliflower, chopped

1 cup of celery, chopped

¼ tsp of turmeric, ground

Preparation:

Wash the asparagus under cold running water. Trim off the woody ends and chop into bite-sized pieces. Set aside.

Wash the cucumber and cut into thin slices. Fill the measuring cup and reserve the rest in the refrigerator.

Wash the cauliflower and trim off the outer leaves. Chop into small pieces and fill the measuring cup. Reserve the rest for later.

Wash the celery and chop into bite-sized pieces. Set aside.

Now, combine asparagus, cucumber, cauliflower, and celery in a juicer and process until juiced. Transfer to a serving glass and stir in the turmeric.

Serve immediately.

Nutrition information per serving: Kcal: 52, Protein: 6.1g, Carbs: 15.4g, Fats: 0.7g

37.   Salted Avocado Juice

Ingredients:

1 cup of avocado, cubed

1 cup of celery, chopped

3 large radishes, chopped

1 small zucchini, sliced

1 cup of cucumber, sliced

¼ tsp of salt

1 oz of water

Preparation:

Peel the avocado and cut in half. Remove the pit and cut into small cubes. Fill the measuring cup and reserve the rest for later.

Wash the celery and chop it into bite-sized pieces. Set aside.

Wash the radishes and cut into small pieces. Set aside.

Wash the zucchini and cut into thin slices. Set aside.

Wash the cucumber and cut into thin slices. Fill the

measuring cup and reserve the rest for later. Set aside.

Now, combine avocado, celery, radishes, zucchini, and cucumber in a juicer and process until juiced. Transfer to a serving glass and stir in the salt and water.

Serve cold.

Nutrition information per serving: Kcal: 235, Protein: 5.6g, Carbs: 22.3g, Fats: 22.6g

38.   Kiwi Apple Juice

Ingredients:

2 whole kiwis, peeled and halved

1 medium-sized Granny Smith's apple, cored

3 whole apricots, chopped

1 large banana, chunked

Preparation:

Peel the kiwi and cut lengthwise in half. Set aside.

Wash the apple and cut lengthwise in half. Remove the core and cut into bite-sized pieces. Set aside.

Wash the apricots and cut in half. Remove the pits and cut into small pieces. Set aside.

Peel the banana and cut into small chunks. Set aside.

Now, combine kiwi, apple, apricots, and banana in a juicer and process until juiced. Transfer to a serving glass and add some ice.

Serve immediately.

Nutrition information per serving: Kcal: 313, Protein: 5.4g, Carbs: 91g, Fats: 1.9g

39.   Kale Parsley Juice

Ingredients:

1 cup of kale, chopped

2 cups of parsley, chopped

1 whole grapefruit, peeled

1 cup of watermelon, diced

2 oz of water

Preparation:

Wash the kale and parsley under cold running water. Torn with hands and set aside.

Peel the grapefruit and cut into small pieces. Set aside.

Cut the watermelon lengthwise. For one cup, you will need about 1 large wedge. Peel and cut into chunks. Remove the seeds and set aside. Reserve the rest of the melon for some other juices.

Now, process kale, parsley, grapefruit, watermelon in a juicer. Transfer to serving glasses and stir in the water.

Add some ice and serve immediately.

Nutrition information per serving: Kcal: 161, Protein: 6.4g, Carbs: 45.6g, Fats: 1.5g

40.   Ginger Pepper Juice

Ingredients:

¼ tsp of ginger, ground

1 large red bell pepper, chopped

1 cup of cauliflower, chopped

1 cup of Brussels sprouts, halved

2 oz of water

Preparation:

Trim off the outer leaves of a cauliflower. Wash it and cut into small pieces. Fill the measuring cup and reserve the rest in the refrigerator.

Wash the Brussels sprouts and trim off the wilted layers. Cut each in half and fill the measuring cup. Set aside.

Wash the bell pepper and cut lengthwise in half. Remove the seeds and the top stem. Cut into small pieces and set aside.

Now, combine pepper, cauliflower, and Brussels sprouts in a juicer and process until juiced. Transfer to a serving glass and stir in the water and ginger.

Serve immediately.

Nutrition information per serving: Kcal: 106, Protein: 9.6g, Carbs: 30.9g, Fats: 1.3g

41.   Coconut Kale Juice

Ingredients:

1 cup of fresh kale, chopped

1 oz of coconut water

1 large banana, peeled and chunked

1 small Granny Smith's apple, cored

1 cup of Brussels sprouts, halved

¼ tsp of ginger, ground

Preparation:

Wash the kale thoroughly under cold running water and slightly drain. Chop into small pieces and set aside.

Peel the banana and cut into small chunks. Set aside.

Wash the apple and cut in half. Remove the core and cut into bite-sized pieces. Set aside.

Wash the Brussels sprouts and remove the outer wilted layers. Cut each in half and set aside.

Now, combine kale, banana, apple, and Brussels sprouts in a juicer and process until juiced. Transfer to a serving glass and stir in the coconut water and ginger.

Add some ice and serve immediately.

Nutrition information per serving: Kcal: 223, Protein: 7.9g, Carbs: 64.4g, Fats: 1.6g

42.   Lemon Beet Juice

Ingredients:

1 whole lemon, peeled

1 cup of beets, sliced

1 cup of raspberries

1 medium-sized pear, chopped

1 oz of water

Preparation:

Peel the lemon and cut lengthwise in half. Set aside.

Wash the beets and trim off the green parts. Cut into thin slices and fill the measuring cup. Reserve the rest for later.

Rinse well the raspberries using a small colander. Drain and set aside.

Wash the pear and cut in half. Remove the core and cut into bite-sized pieces. Set aside.

Now, combine lemon, beets, raspberries, and pear in a juicer and process until juiced. Transfer to a serving glass and stir in the water.

Refrigerate for 5 minutes before serving.

Nutrition information per serving: Kcal: 165, Protein: 4.9g, Carbs: 60.2g, Fats: 1.4g

43.   Blackberry Pineapple Juice

Ingredients:

1 cup of blackberries

1 cup of pineapple, chunked

1 whole lime, peeled

1 large banana, sliced

2 oz of water

Preparation:

Place the blackberries in a small colander and wash under cold running water. Slightly drain and set aside.

Using a sharp paring knife, cut the top of the pineapple. Gently remove all hard skin and slice it into thin slices. Fill the measuring cup and reserve the rest for later.

Peel the banana and cut into thin slices. Set aside.

Peel the lime and cut lengthwise in half. Set aside.

Now, combine blackberries, pineapple, banana, and lime in a juicer. Process until well juiced. Transfer to a serving glass and add some ice before serving.

Enjoy!

Nutrition information per serving: Kcal: 222, Protein: 4.5g, Carbs: 70.2g, Fats: 1.4g

44.   Watercress Rosemary Juice

Ingredients:

1 cup of watercress, torn

1 rosemary sprig, finely chopped

1 medium whole tomato, chopped

1 large red bell pepper, chopped

1 oz of water

Preparation:

Wash the watercress thoroughly under cold running water. Slightly drain and torn with hands into small pieces. Set aside.

Wash the tomato and place in a small bowl. Chop into small pieces and make sure to reserve the tomato juice while cutting. Set aside.

Wash the bell pepper and cut lengthwise in half. Remove the seeds and chop into small pieces. Set aside.

Now, combine watercress, bell pepper, and tomato in a juicer and process until juiced. Transfer to a serving glass and stir in the water and reserved tomato juice.

Sprinkle with rosemary and serve immediately.

Enjoy!

Nutrition information per serving: Kcal: 56, Protein: 3.5g, Carbs: 15.1g, Fats: 0.7g

45.   Carrot Apple Juice

Ingredients:

1 large carrot, sliced

1 small Red Delicious apple, cored

1 cup of celery, chopped

1 whole lemon, peeled

¼ tsp ginger, ground

1 oz of water

Preparation:

Wash and peel the carrot. Cut into small slices and set aside.

Wash the apple and cut in half. Remove the core and cut into bite-sized pieces. Set aside.

Wash the celery and cut into small pieces. Set aside.

Peel the lemon and cut lengthwise in half. Set aside.

Now, combine carrot, apple, celery, and lemon in a juicer and process until juiced. Transfer to a serving glass and stir in the water and ginger. If you like, add some crushed ice.

Serve immediately.

Nutrition information per serving: Kcal: 105, Protein: 2.4g, Carbs: 32.8g, Fats: 0.7g

46.   Spinach Swiss Chard Juice

Ingredients:

1 cup of fresh spinach, chopped

1 cup of Swiss chard, torn

1 cup of cucumber, sliced

1 cup of fresh kale, chopped

¼ tsp of ginger, ground

1 oz of water

Preparation:

Combine spinach, kale, and Swiss chard in a large colander. Rinse under cold running water and slightly drain. Chop all into small pieces and set aside.

Wash the cucumber and cut into thin slices. Fill the measuring cup and reserve the rest in the refrigerator.

Now, combine spinach, Swiss chard, cucumber, and kale in a juicer and process until well juiced. Transfer to a serving glass and stir in the ginger and water.

Refrigerate before serving.

Enjoy!

Nutrition information per serving: Kcal: 63, Protein: 9.9g, Carbs: 16.7g, Fats: 1.6g

47.   Spinach Tomato Juice

Ingredients:

1 cup of fresh spinach, torn

1 medium-sized tomato, chopped

1 cup of purple cabbage, chopped

1 cup of beets, sliced

1 large red bell pepper, chopped

¼ tsp of salt

Preparation:

Combine spinach and cabbage in a large colander. Rinse thoroughly under cold running water and drain. Torn into small pieces and set aside.

Wash the tomato and chop into small pieces. Set aside.

Wash the beets and trim off the green parts. Peel and cut into thin slices and fill the measuring cup. Reserve the rest for later.

Wash the bell pepper and cut lengthwise in half. Remove the stem and seeds. Cut into small pieces and set aside.

Now, combine spinach, tomatoes, cabbage, beets, and bell

pepper in a juicer and process until juiced. Transfer to a serving glass and stir in the salt.

Serve immediately.

Nutrition information per serving: Kcal: 134, Protein: 11.5g, Carbs: 39.1g, Fats: 1.8g

48.   Carrot Fennel Juice

Ingredients:

1 medium-sized carrot, sliced

1 medium-sized fennel bulb

1 small ginger knob, peeled

½ cup of cabbage, torn

2 oz of water

Preparation:

Wash and peel the carrot. Cut into thin slices and set aside.

Wash the fennel and trim off the green ends. Using a sharp paring knife, remove the outer layer. Cut into small pieces and set aside.

Peel the ginger knob and cut into small pieces. Set aside.

Wash the cabbage thoroughly and torn into small pieces. Set aside.

Now, combine carrot, fennel, ginger, and cabbage in a juicer and process until juiced. Transfer to a serving glass and stir in the water. Refrigerate before serving.

Enjoy!

Nutrition information per serving: Kcal: 72, Protein: 4g, Carbs: 25.9g, Fats: 0.7g

MEALS

1.   Grapefruit Broccoli Smoothie

Ingredients:

1 cup of broccoli, halved

1 medium-sized banana, sliced

½ grapefruit, peeled and chopped

1 tbsp of sesame seeds

1 cup of water

Preparation:

Combine all ingredients in a food processor. Blend until smooth mixture and transfer to a serving glasses. Refrigerate 30 minutes before serving.

Nutrition information per serving: Kcal: 265, Protein: 7.4g, Carbs: 55.3g, Fats: 6.7g

2.   Potato Casserole

Ingredients:

6 large potatoes, peeled and halved

2 cups of broccoli, halved

1 cup of cheddar cheese, shredded

1 cup of green onions, chopped

1 tbsp of olive oil

¼ tsp of salt

¼ tsp of black pepper, ground

Preparation:

Preheat the oven to a 350°F.

Place the potatoes in a large pot of boiling water. Cook until fork-tender and remove from the heat. Remove from the heat and drain. Leave it to cool for 10 minutes. In a separate pot, place the broccoli into a boiling process and cook until soften. Remove from the heat and drain. Set aside.

Halve the potatoes and place them into a greased baking dish. Now, make another layer with halved broccoli. Top with shredded cheese and put it in the oven. Bake for 25 minutes. Remove from the oven and sprinkle with chopped spring onions. Leave it to cool for few minutes and cut into desired portions.

Nutrition information per serving: Kcal: 351, Protein: 13.2g, Carbs: 60.7g, Fats: 6.4g

3.   Garbanzo Salad

Ingredients:

2 cups of garbanzo beans, pre-cooked

2 cups of kidney beans, pre-cooked

3 cups of Iceberg lettuce, shredded

1 large tomato, chopped

1 medium-sized cucumber, sliced

1 small avocado, peeled, pitted and chopped

1 cup of yogurt, fat free

1 garlic clove, crushed

¼ tsp of cumin, ground

Preparation:

Place garbanzo and kidney beans in a pot of boiling water. Cook until soften. Remove from the heat and let it cool for a while.

Now, combine beans, tomato, and cucumber in a large salad bowl. Set aside.

Meanwhile, combine avocado, yogurt, cumin, and garlic in

a food processor. Blend until smooth and drizzle over the salad.

Place a handful of shredded lettuce on a serving plate and top with 2-3 tablespoons of previously made salad.

Serve immediately.

Nutrition information per serving: Kcal: 171, Protein: 8.6g, Carbs: 28.8g, Fats: 3.7g

4.   Oven Baked Rice with Spring Onions

Ingredients:

2 cups of long grain rice

4 tbsp of extra virgin olive oil

1 tsp of salt

3 whole eggs

5 spring onions, finely chopped

½ tsp of black pepper, freshly ground

Preparation:

Preheat the oven to 350°F.

Use a package instructions to prepare the rice. Set aside.

In a medium-sized skillet heat up two tablespoons of olive oil and add onions. Stir fry for 3-4 minutes. Meanwhile, beat the eggs and pour into skillet. Cook for two minutes, remove from the heat and combine with rice.

Spread the remaining oil in a small casserole dish. Add rice mixture, salt, and pepper. Bake for 20 minutes.

Serve warm.

Instead of oven, you can prepare this dish in a large wok pan. Simply stir-fry the cooked rice until lightly crispy. Serve.

Nutrition Information per serving: Kcal: 409, Protein: 8.9g, Carbs: 60g, Fats: 14.3g

5. Watermelon Salad

Ingredients:

6 cups of watermelon, cut into bite-sized pieces

2 tbsp of balsamic vinegar

½ small red onion, sliced

1 tbsp of fresh mint, roughly chopped

½ tsp of salt

Preparation:

Place the onion into a medium pot. Pour water enough to cover it and add a pinch of salt. Set aside for 15 minutes. Drain well and transfer to a large salad bowl.

Add watermelon chops and drizzle with vinegar. Give it a good stir and top with fresh mint leaves.

Nutrition information per serving: Kcal: 53, Protein: 0.9g, Carbs: 12.5g, Fats: 0.3g

6. Poached Salmon

Ingredients:

1 lb of wild salmon fillets, skinless and boneless

1 tbsp of fresh dill, finely chopped

1 large onion, sliced

2 small carrots, sliced

2 tbsp of lemon juice

2 bay leaves

4 cups of water

Preparation:

Preheat the oven to 350°F.

Pour water in a large skillet. Bring it to a boil and add dill, carrots, onion, lemon juice, and bay leaves. Cook for about 2-3 minutes and remove from the heat. Set aside.

Meanwhile, place the salmon fillets into a large baking sheet. Pour the previously prepared liquid. Cover with a lid and place it in the oven. Bake for 20 minutes, or until set. Remove from the heat and leave it to cool for a while.

Serve.

Nutrition information per serving: Kcal: 239, Protein: 24.5g, Carbs: 6.3g, Fats: 5.2g

7.   Ginger Dates Smoothie

Ingredients:

1 cup of spinach, chopped

½ medium-sized avocado, pitted, peeled, and cubed

3 dates, pitted and chopped

1 tbsp of lemon juice

1 tbsp of fresh ginger, grated

Preparation:

Combine all ingredients in a food processor. Blend until nicely smooth. Transfer to a serving glasses and refrigerate for 15 minutes. For extra thickness, refrigerate more.

Nutrition information per serving: Kcal: 389, Protein: 5.2g, Carbs: 48.8g, Fats: 21.2g

8.   Warm Broccoli Soup

Ingredients:

2oz fresh broccoli

2oz Brussel sprouts

A handful of fresh parsley, finely chopped

1 tsp of dry thyme

1 tbsp of fresh lemon juice

¼ tsp of sea salt

Preparation:

Place the broccoli in a deep pot and pour enough water to cover. Bring it to a boil and cook until tender. Remove from the heat and drain.

Transfer to a food processor. Add fresh parsley, thyme, and about 1 cup of water. Pulse until smooth mixture. Return to a pot and add some more water. Bring it to a boil and cook for several minutes, over a minimum temperature. Season with salt and add fresh lemon juice. Serve warm.

Nutrition information per serving: Kcal: 50, Protein: 3.7g, Carbs: 9.9g, Fats: 0.6g

9.   Stuffed Tomatoes

Ingredients:

10 oz of spinach, chopped

4 medium-sized tomatoes

½ cup of Mozzarella cheese, crumbled

½ cup of Parmesan cheese, grated

1 small onion, finely chopped

2 tbsp of fresh parsley, finely chopped

¼ tsp of salt

¼ tsp of black pepper, ground

Preparation:

Preheat the oven to 350°F.

Place spinach in a pot of boiling water. Cook for 2 minutes, or until soften. Remove from the heat and drain well. Set aside.

Hollow the tomatoes and reserve the pulp. Chop it into a small pieces and add it to spinach. Stir in the cheeses and toss well to combine. Spoon in the mixture into tomatoes. Place stuffed tomatoes in a large baking sheet. Place it in the oven and bake for about 6-7 minutes. Remove from the heat and leave it to cool for a while.

Nutrition information per serving: Kcal: 159, Protein: 13.2g, Carbs: 15.6g, Fats: 7.3g

10. Brown Rice Mushroom Risotto

Ingredients:

1 cup of brown rice

1 cup of button mushrooms, sliced

½ medium-sized onion, finely chopped

3 spring onions, sliced

3 tbsp of extra virgin olive oil

½ tsp of salt

1 tsp of dry marjoram

Preparation:

Place the rice in a deep pot. Add 2 cups of water and bring it to a boil. Reduce the heat and cook until the water evaporates. Stir occasionally. Set aside.

Heat up one tablespoon of olive oil over a medium-high heat. Add chopped onion and stir-fry for 3-4 minutes, stirring constantly. Now add the mushrooms and continue to cook until the water evaporates.

Stir in the remaining olive oil, rice, spring onions, salt, and marjoram. Add one cup of water and continue to cook for another 10 minutes.

Serve warm.

Nutrition information per serving: Kcal: 243, Protein: 16.4g, Carbs: 24.5g, Fats: 11.3g

11.   Peanut Butter Smoothie

Ingredients:

1 medium-sized banana, sliced

½ cup of Greek yogurt

1 tbsp of cinnamon, ground

1 tbsp of peanut butter

1 tbsp of coconut flour

Preparation:

Combine all ingredients in a food processor. Blend all until smooth mixture. Transfer to a serving glass and refrigerate for 1 hour before serving.

Nutrition information per serving: Kcal: 216, Protein: 5.6g, Carbs: 35.6g, Fats: 8.5g

12.   Black Beans & Squash Stew

Ingredients:

1 medium-sized butternut squash, peeled and chopped

4 cups of black beans, canned

4 large tomatoes, blended

1 small onion, sliced

1 garlic clove, minced

4 medium-sized bell peppers, chopped

1 tsp of cumin, ground

1 tsp of dried oregano, minced

1 tbsp of olive oil

¼ tsp of black pepper, ground

¼ tsp of salt

Preparation:

Place squash in a pot of boiling water and cook for 10 minutes, or until fork-tender. Drain well and set aside.

Preheat the oil in a large pot over a medium-high temperature. Add onions and stir-fry for 5 minutes, or until translucent. Add beans, garlic, peppers, cumin, and oregano and stir.

Meanwhile, place tomatoes in a food processor and blend until smooth mixture. Transfer to a pot and give it a good stir. Bring to a boil and reduce the heat to low. Add squash, stir once, and cover with a lid. Cook for about 20-25 minutes and remove from the heat. Sprinkle with some salt and pepper to taste.

Serve warm.

Nutrition information per serving: Kcal: 201, Protein: 8.2g, Carbs: 40.3g, Fats: 3.7g

13.   Curry Veggies Salad

Ingredients:

1 lb of broccoli, halved

1 cup of sour cream, fat-free

2 large tomatoes, wedged

1 tsp of curry powder

¼ tsp of dry mustard

½ cup of skim milk

5 Romaine lettuce leaves

Preparation:

Place broccoli in a pot of boiling water and cook until soften. Remove from the heat and drain well. Transfer to a serving bowl and set aside to cool for 5 minutes.

Meanwhile, combine, milk, sour cream, curry, and mustard in a mixing bowl. Toss well to combine and pour over the broccoli. Add tomato wedges and stir well.

Place lettuce leaves on a serving plate and spoon the salad onto it. Refrigerate for 2 hours to allow flavors to mingle.

Nutrition information per serving: Kcal: 109, Protein: 3.8g, Carbs: 11.4g, Fats: 2.2g

14. Brown Rice Pudding with Raspberries and Chia Seeds

Ingredients:

¾ cup of brown rice

1 cup of rice milk

¼ cup of honey

1 tbsp of almond butter

¼ tsp of salt

½ cup of raspberries

¼ cup of walnuts

2 tbsp of chia seeds

Preparation:

Bring 2 cups of water to a boil. Add rice and reduce the heat. Cover and cook for about 15 minutes.

Now add one cup of rice milk, honey, almond butter, and salt. Continue to cook for five more minutes. Remove from the heat and cool for a while.

Top with fresh raspberries, walnuts, and chia seeds. Serve.

Nutrition information per serving: Kcal: 240, Protein: 5.7g, Carbs: 36.7g, Fats: 8.4g

15.   Crispy Cauliflower Sliders

Ingredients:

1 cup of fresh button mushrooms

3 tbsp of flax seeds plus 9 tbsp of water

¾ cup of chia seeds

¾ cup of brown rice

¾ cup of buckwheat bread crumbs

1 tsp of tarragon

1 tsp of parsley

1 tsp of garlic powder

1 cup of chopped spinach

Preparation:

Pour 1 cup of water in a small saucepan. Bring it to boil and cook rice until it's slightly sticky. This should take about 10 minutes.

At the same time, cook chia seeds until soft in a separate pot. Finely chop mushrooms. Thoroughly rinse spinach. Mix all the ingredients together in a large bowl. Put the bowl into the fridge to chill for 15 to 30 minutes.

Take mixture out of the fridge and form into patties. Make sure cooking surfaces are cleaned and greased before adding patties to prevent them from sticking. Fry each piece on a medium temperature for about 5 minutes on both side.

Nutrition information per serving: Kcal: 220, Protein: 6.1g, Carbs: 40.1g, Fats: 3.6g

16. Tomato Strawberry Smoothie

Ingredients:

½ cantaloupe, peeled and chopped

1 cup of orange juice

1 cup of strawberries, halved

1 medium-sized tomato, chopped

Preparation:

Combine all ingredients in a blender. Add few ice cubes and blend until nicely smooth. Transfer to a serving glass and serve immediately!

Nutrition information per serving: Kcal: 253, Protein: 5.3g, Carbs: 62.4g, Fats: 1.2g

17.   Ginger Quinoa Porridge

Ingredients:

1/2 cup of orange juice

1 tsp of fresh ginger, grated

½ cup of dates, pitted and chopped

1 cup of white quinoa, pre-cooked

½ cup of dried apricots, chopped

1 tsp of fresh orange zest, grated

1 tsbp of toasted almonds, chopped

¼ tsp of cinnamon, ground

Preparation:

Place quinoa in a pot of boiling water. Cook for 3 minutes and reduce the heat to low. Cook for another 10 minutes or until soften and fluffy. Add all other ingredients except almonds and give it a good stir. Remove from the heat and set aside for 10 minutes to cool. Top with chopped almonds and serve.

Nutrition information per serving: Kcal: 171, Protein: 5.2g, Carbs: 32.5g, Fats: 4.7g

18.   Creamy Pumpkin Soup

Ingredients:

3 lbs of pumpkin, peeled and cubed

2 small onions, sliced

5 cups of chicken broth

2 cups of skim milk

3 tbsp of Greek yogurt

2 tbsp of pumpkin seeds

1 garlic clove, minced

1 tsp of vegetable oil

¼ tsp of salt

¼ tsp of black pepper, ground

Preparation:

Preheat the oil in a large nonstick saucepan over a medium-high temperature. Add onions and stir-fry until soften. Add vegetable broth, pumpkin cubes, milk, sage, and garlic. Bring it to a boil and reduce the heat to low. Cover with a lid and cook for 35 minutes. Remove from the heat and set aside to cool for 10 minutes.

Transfer the mixture into a food processor. Blend until nicely creamy mixture. Transfer to a serving bowl or previously used saucepan. Add a pinch of salt and pepper to taste and stir well.

Serve warm.

Nutrition information per serving: Kcal: 191, Protein: 4.3g, Carbs: 27.7g, Fats: 4.1g

19.   Nutmeg Fruit Smoothie

Ingredients:

2 large oranges, peeled and wedged

2 medium-sized apples, wedged

1 small mango, peeled, pitted and chopped

1 small carrot, sliced

½ tsp of nutmeg

1 tsp of cinnamon, ground

1 tbsp of honey

½ cup of water

Preparation:

Combine all ingredients in a food processor. Blend until smooth and transfer to a serving glasses. Refrigerate 30 minutes before serving.

Nutrition information per serving: Kcal: 316, Protein: 3.6g, Carbs: 79.5g, Fats: 1.8g

20.　Zuchini Lasagna

Ingredients:

1 medium-sized zuchinni, peeled and chopped

2 oz of Parmesan cheese, grated

2 oz of cottage cheese, crumbled

2 oz of Mozarella cheese, grated

8 oz of lasagna noodles, pre-cooked

2 cups of tomato sauce

1 small onion, sliced

1 garlic clove, minced

¼ tsp of oregano, ground

2 tsp of dried basil, ground

½ tsp of Cayenne pepper, ground

¼ tsp of salt

Preparation:

Preheat the oven to 370 °F.

Place zucchini in a pot of boiling water. Cook until fork-tender and remove from the heat to cool for 5 minutes. Drain well and slice into small bite-sized pieces. Set aside.

Combine all cheeses in a mixing bowl. Pour in the tomato sauce and stir well.

Grease a large baking dish with some oil. Spread the cheese and tomato mixture and make a first layer. Now, add one layer of noodles, then one layer of zucchini slices. Repeat layering process until left out of ingredients. Add some extra cheese and 1 tablespoon of tomato sauce on top. Sprinkle with Cayenne pepper for extra flavor.

Cover with foil and put it in the oven. Bake for 30 minutes and remove from the oven to cool.

Cut into portions and serve warm.

Nutrition information per serving: Kcal: 275, Protein: 18.3g, Carbs: 41.3g, Fats: 5.4g

21. Leafy Detox Smoothie

Ingredients:

¼ cup of roasted almonds, finely chopped

¼ cup of baby spinach, finely chopped

¼ cup of arugula

1 tbsp of almond butter

½ tsp of ground turmeric

1 cup of rice milk

A handful of ice cubes

Preparation:

Toss all the ingredients in a blender. Pulse to combine.

Nutrition information per serving: Kcal: 181, Protein: 4.6g, Carbs: 17.1g, Fats: 11.5g

22. Turkey & Mushrooms Stew

Ingredients:

1 lb of turkey breasts, skinless and boneless

5 oz of button mushrooms, chopped

2 garlic cloves, minced

1 tbsp of fresh parsley, finely chopped

1 tbsp of honey, raw

½ tsp of salt

¼ tsp of black pepper, ground

Preparation:

Combine all ingredients except honey in a slow cooker. Pour water enough to cover all ingredients. Cover with a lid and cook for 7 hours. Remove from the heat and let it stand for 20 minutes. Open the lid and let it cool for 10 minutes and then stir in honey.

Nutrition information per serving: Kcal: 116, Protein: 16.5g, Carbs: 8.8g, Fats: 1.7g

23. Quinoa Muffins

Ingredients:

1.5 cups of quinoa flour

0.5 cup of buckwheat flour

3 tbsp of almond butter

1 cup of almond milk

½ cup of honey

1 tsp of baking powder

½ tsp of salt

2 tbsp of raw cocoa

2 tbsp of flax seed plus 6 tbsp of water

1 tsp organic vanilla extract

1 tsp lemon zest

Preparation:

Preheat oven to 325 degrees. Line one 6-cup muffin tins with paper liners.

Combine all dry ingredients in a large bowl. Gently whisk in almond milk, almond butter, and beat well on high. Add flax seed, water, lemon zest, and reduce the speed to low. Continue beating until well incorporated.

Using a spoon or ice cream scoop, divide the mixture evenly among the tins. Bake for 20-30 or until the toothpick inserted into the middle comes out clean.

Nutrition information per serving: Kcal: 182, Protein: 4.2g, Carbs: 12.3g, Fats: 14.6g

24.   Pineapple Smoothie

Ingredients:

1 cup of pineapple, canned

1 cup of Greek yogurt

½ medium-sized banana, sliced

½ cup of strawberries, halved

1 tsp of vanilla extract

Preparation:

Combine all ingredients in a food processor. Blend until smooth. Add few ice cubes and re-blend. Transfer to a serving glasses and serve immediately.

Nutrition information per serving: Kcal: 122, Protein: 6.3g, Carbs: 24.3g, Fats: 0.8g

25.   Rice Yogurt with Fresh Plums and Chia Seeds

Ingredients:

2 tbsp of chia seeds, soaked

½ cup of almond milk

½ cup of rice yogurt

1.5oz quinoa

½ cup of water

2 medium-sized plums, sliced

1 tbsp of honey

Preparation:

Combine the water and almond milk in a medium sized saucepan. Bring it to a boil and add quinoa. Reduce the heat and cook for about 20 minutes, or until all the liquid evaporates.

Transfer the cooked quinoa to a bowl. Stir in the rice yogurt and chia seeds.

Top with sliced plums and serve.

Nutrition information per serving: Kcal: 241, Protein: 4.9g, Carbs: 25g, Fats: 15.8g

26. Rice with Pecans

Ingredients:

10 oz of brown rice

1 small onion, chopped

1 cup of fresh celery, finely chopped

1 medium-sized bell pepper, chopped

2 tbsp of pecans, roughly chopped

1 tbsp of dried sage, ground

2 tbsp of vegetable oil

1 cup of chicken broth, unsalted

12 oz of water

¼ tsp of salt

Preparation:

Combine chicken broth and water in a large pot and bring it to a boil. Add rice and give it a good stir. Reduce the heat to low and cover with a lid. Cook for about 15-20 minutes. Remove from the heat and let it stand for 5-6 minutes to cool. Set aside.

Preheat the oil in a large nonstick pan over a low temperature. Add onions and stir-fry until translucent. Stir in the celery and cook for 5 minutes more. Now, add all ingredients except pecans. Add previously cooked rice and give it a good stir to combine. Cook for 1 minute more. Remove from the heat and serve warm.

Nutrition information per serving: Kcal: 140, Protein: 2.8g, Carbs: 22.3g, Fats: 5.7g

27.   Steamed Chicken

Ingredients:

1 lb of chicken legs, cut into bite-sized pieces

¼ tsp of ginger, ground

2 ginger sticks, 2 inches long

1 tbsp of garlic, minced

1 cup of spring onions

¼ tsp of salt

3 tbsp of olive oil

Preparation:

Rub the chicken with ginger and salt. Set aside to marinate for 10 minutes.

Take a large baking sheet and place ginger sticks and garlic at the bottom. Spread the chicken chops evenly over it.

Steam for about 30-35 minutes on high temperature. Remove from the heat to cool completely. Place it into a plastic bags and transfer to cold water.

Now, remove the bones and arrange into a serving portion. Meanwhile, combine onions, oil, and a pinch of salt into a mixing bowl. Top over the chicken.

Serve with some cooked vegetables, such as broccoli, cauliflower, etc.

Nutrition information per serving: Kcal: 254, Protein: 26.7g, Carbs: 3.2g, Fats: 15.3g

28.   Rice Casserole

Ingredients:

2 large broccoli crowns, chopped

7oz brussel sprouts, halved

1 cup of quinoa, rinsed

4 cups of homemade vegetable broth

2 small onions, finely chopped

1 cup of sour cashew cream

2 tsp dry thyme

4 tbsp of extra virgin olive oil

Salt and pepper to taste

Preparation:

Preheat the oven to 400 degrees.

In a large saucepan, combine quinoa with vegetable broth and dry thyme. Add some salt and pepper to taste and bring it to a boil. Reduce the heat and cook until the liquid is absorbed, about 12-15 minutes. Remove from the heat and set aside.

Heat up the olive oil in a large saucepan. Add onions and stir-fry for 2-3 minutes, or until translucent. Now add chopped broccoli and brussel sprouts. Continue to cook for ten more minutes, or until the broccoli and brussel sprouts are tender-crisp.

Combine the broccoli mixture with quinoa in a large bowl. Add cashew cream and stir well. Place in a lightly oiled shallow casserole dish. Bake for about 20 minutes, or until the top is lightly charred and crisp.

Serve!

Nutrition information per serving: Kcal: 352, Protein: 13g, Carbs: 36.3g, Fats: 18.2g

29.   Quinoa Artichoke Soup

Ingredients:

14 oz of artichoke hearts, canned

4 cups of vegetable broth, unsalted

1 cup of white quinoa, pre-cooked

1 small onion, sliced

2 tbsp of fresh lemon juice

1 garlic clove, minced

1 cup of skim milk

1 tsp of brown sugar

¼ tsp of salt

¼ tsp of black pepper, ground

Preparation:

Place quinoa in a large nonstick pan over a medium-high temperature. Cook for 5 minutes, stirring constantly. Remove from the heat and transfer quinoa in another bowl. Reserve the pan.

Preheat the oil in the same pan and add onions and garlic.

Stir-fry until translucent. Add vegetable broth, lemon juice, and previously toasted quinoa.

Bring it to a boil and reduce the temperature to low. Cover with a lid and simmer for 15 minutes, or until tender.

Now, add artichokes and cook for another 5-7 minutes. Remove from the heat and use kitchen hand mixer to puree the soup.

Return the heat and add sugar and milk. Stir constantly for 2 minutes. Remove from the heat and sprinkle with salt and pepper to taste. Serve warm.

Nutrition information per serving: Kcal: 191, Protein: 10.3g, Carbs: 27.4g, Fats: 5.3g

30.　　Quick Maple Pecan Oatmeal

Ingredients:

2 cups of rolled oats

2 tbsp of coconut flour

½ cup of pecans, roughly chopped

3 tbsp of raisins, chopped

3 tbsp of maple syrup

1 tbsp of honey

1 tsp of cinnamon, ground

1 tsp of vanilla extract

Preparation:

Use package instructions to cook oats. Remove from the heat and let it cool. Transfer to a large bowl and add all other ingredients.

Stir all well to combine and serve wiht some extra nuts if you like.

Nutrition information per serving: Kcal: 313, Protein: 5.6g, Carbs: 63.5g, Fats: 3.6g

31. Asparagus and Leek Soup

Ingredients:

1 lb of fresh wild asparagus, trimmed and chopped

1 cup of leeks, chopped

2 cups of vegetable broth, unsalted

2 medium-sized potatoes, peeled and chopped

2 garlic cloves, minced

1 tbsp of olive oil

½ cup of green beans, pre-cooked

1 tbsp of fresh parsley, finely chopped

2 cups of skim milk

¼ tsp of lemon juice

¼ tsp of salt

¼ tsp of black pepper, ground

Preparation:

Preheat the oil in a large skillet over a medium-low temperature. Add leeks and cook for about 5-7 minutes, or until soften. Add garlic and cook for another minute. Stir constantly.

Pour in the vegetable broth. Increase the temperature to high and add potatoes. Cover with a lid and cook until potatoes are fork-tender. Add asparagus and green beans. Cook for another 4-5 minutes. Remove from the heat and stir in all other ingredients. Stir all well and transfer to a food processor or blender. Blend until nicely smooth creamy mixture. Return the mixture to the skillet.

Cook for 15 minutes on low heat and remove from the heat. Let it cool and serve.

Nutrition information per serving: Kcal: 190, Protein: 8.7g, Carbs: 28.8g, Fats: 4.7g

32.   Sweet Rice Noodles

Ingredients:

14oz rice noodles

2 tbsp of olive oil

2 tsp ground turmeric

2 cups of coconut milk

½ cup of sour cashew cream

2 tbsp of almond butter

¼ cup of fresh lime juice

A handful of toasted cashews

1 tsp of powdered honey

1 medium-sized onion, finely chopped

1 tbsp fresh ginger, grated

Preparation:

Soak the noodles for five minutes. Drain and set aside.

Heat up the olive oil and add ground turmeric. Briefly cook for about a minute. Now add coconut milk and bring it to a boil. Reduce the heat and add almond butter, cashew cream, fresh lime juice, cashews, honey, chopped onion, and fresh ginger. Continue to cook for about five minutes.

Add noodles and mix well. Cover and allow it to warm up. Serve.

Nutrition information per serving: Kcal: 342, Protein: 3.9g, Carbs: 24.7g, Fats: 27g

33.   Ice Cappuccino Smoothie

Ingredients:

1 tsp of instant espresso powder

1 tbsp of liquid chocolate

1 cup of skim milk

¼ tsp of cinnamon

1 tsp of honey

Preparation:

Combine all ingredients in a blender except cinnamon. Blend until smooth. Add few ice cubes, and re-blend. Transfer to a serving glass. Sprinkle with cinnamon and serve.

Nutrition information per serving: Kcal: 169, Protein: 8.7g, Carbs: 24.3g, Fats: 3.1g

34.   Almond Yogurt with Nuts

Ingredients:

1 cup of almond yogurt

A handful of walnuts, chopped

1 tbsp of chia seeds

1 tbsp of homemade fig spread

Preparation:

Combine one cup of almond yogurt with chia seeds. Top with chopped nuts and fig spread. Serve immediately!

Nutrition information per serving: Kcal: 192, Protein: 6.1g, Carbs: 33g, Fats: 7.9g

35.   Spring Purple Salad

Ingredients:

½ medium red cabbage head

2 large spring onions, sliced

2 medium-sized carrots, sliced

¼ cup of extra virgin olive oil

2 tbsp of fresh lemon juice

½ tsp of sea salt

½ tsp of freshly ground black pepper

Preparation:

Cut cabbage in large pieces and place it in a food processor. Pulse quickly until chopped roughly. Be careful not to process too much.

Combine the cabbage with sliced carrots and spring onions. Toss with olive oil, lemon juice, sea salt, and black pepper.

Nutrition information per serving: Kcal: 254, Protein: 1.1g, Carbs: 8.5g, Fats: 25.4g

36.   Rosemary Couscous

Ingredients:

1 cup of instant couscous

2 large carrots

½ tsp of dried rosemary

1 cup of green beans, cooked and drained

10 green olives, pitted

1 tbsp of lemon juice

1 tbsp of orange juice

1 tbsp of orange zest

4 tbsp of olive oil

½ tsp of salt

Preparation:

Wash and peel carrots. Cut into thin slices. Heat up 2 tbsp of olive oil in a large pan over medium heat.

Add carrots and cook, stirring constantly. It should be tender after about 10-15 minutes. Add rosemary, green beans, olives and orange juice. Mix well.

Continue to cook and stir occasionally.

Combine lemon juice with 1 cup of water. Add this mixture to a saucepan and mix with 2 tbsp of olive oil, orange zest and salt. Allow it to boil and add couscous. Remove from heat and allow it to stand for about 15 minutes.

Pour these two mixtures into a large bowl and mix well with a tablespoon.

Nutrition information per serving: Kcal: 396, Protein: 1.8g, Carbs: 12.9g, Fats: 28g

37.   Lean Grilled Avocado

Ingredients:

1 large avocado, chopped

¼ cup of water

1 tbsp of ground curry

2 tbsp of olive oil

1 tbsp of tomato sauce

1 tsp of chopped parsley

¼ tsp of red pepper

¼ tsp of sea salt

Preparation:

Heat up olive oil in a large saucepan, over a medium temperature. In a small bowl, combine ground curry, tomato sauce, chopped parsley, red pepper and sea salt. Add water and cook for about 5 minutes, over a medium temperature.

Add chopped avocado, stir well and cook for another few minutes, until all the liquid evaporates. Turn off the heat and cover.

Let it stand for about 15-20 minutes before serving.

Nutrition information per serving: Kcal: 332, Protein: 2.2g, Carbs: 10.2g, Fats: 33g

38.   Turkey Cauliflower Omelet

Ingredients:

1 lb of turkey breast, boneless and skinless

2 lbs of cauliflower, grated

4 garlic cloves, crushed

3 large eggs

1 cup of spring onions, chopped

4 tbsp of olive oil

¼ tsp of sea salt

¼ tsp of black pepper, ground

Preparation:

Squeeze the excessive liquid out of cauliflower and transfer to a large bowl. Set aside.

Preheat the oil in a large saucepan over a medium-high temperature. Add garlic and stir-fry until translucent. Add meat and cook until for about 10-15 minutes, or until almost set. Reduce the heat to low.

Meanwhile, beat the eggs in a mixing bowl nad pour into a saucepan. Stir in grated cauliflower. Add a pinch of salt and pepper to taste. Cook until eggs scrambled, or until cauliflower tender crisp.

Spoon the spring onion and spread over the meat. Cook for another minute and remove from the heat. Add extra salt if necessary.

Serve warm.

Nutrition information per serving: Kcal: 361, Protein: 29.3g, Carbs: 20.1g, Fats: 19.3g

39.   Baked Mushrooms in Tomato Sauce

Ingredients:

1 cup of button mushrooms

1 large tomato

3 tbsp of olive oil

2 cloves of garlic

1 tbsp of fresh basil

Salt and pepper to taste

Preparation:

Wash and peel tomato. Cut in small pieces. Chop garlic and mix with tomato and fresh basil. Heat up the olive oil in a saucepan and put tomato in it. Add ¼ cup of water, mix well and cook for about 15 minutes, on a low temperature, until the water evaporates. Stir constantly. After about 15 minutes, when all the water has evaporated, remove from heat.

Wash and drain mushrooms. Place them in small baking dish and spread tomato sauce over it. Salt and pepper to taste.

Preheat the oven to 300 degrees and bake for about 10-15

minutes.

Nutrition information per serving: Kcal: 209, Protein: 2.1g, Carbs: 5.8g, Fats: 21.4g

40.   Sour potato soup

Ingredients:

1 large potato, peeled and chopped into bite-sized pieces

1 medium-sized onion, peeled and finely chopped

2 small carrots, sliced

4 cups of vegetable broth

A handful of fresh parsley

1 tbsp of apple cider vinegar

1 tsp of salt

½ tsp of pepper

2 tbsp extra virgin olive oil

Preparation:

Heat up the oil in a heavy bottomed saucepan. Add onions and stir-fry until translucent. Now add sliced carrot and potatoes. Continue to cook for five more minutes.

Pour in the vegetable broth, add apple cider, salt, and pepper. Reduce the heat to minimum and cook until potatoes are fork tender.

Serve warm.

Nutrition information per serving: Kcal: 192, Protein: 7.2g, Carbs: 22.3, Fats: 8.5g

41.   Mushroom Salad with Gorgonzola

Ingredients:

1 lb of button mushrooms, chopped

4 oz of Gorgonzola cheese, crumbled

1 bell pepper, roasted, finely chopped

1 cup of Romaine lettuce, chopped

1 cup of sour cream

1 tbsp of mayonnaise

1 tbsp of balsamic vinegar

1 garlic clove, minced

1 tbsp of butter

¼ tsp of salt

¼ tsp of black pepper, ground

Preparation:

Combine cheese, sour cream, vinegar, mayonnaise, red pepper, and garlic in a large mixing bowl. Mash well with fork or use an electric mixer. Sprinkle with some salt and pepper and set aside to allow flavors to mingle.

Melt the butter in a large frying pan over a medium-high temperature. Add mushrooms and cook for 10 minutes, or until set. Stir occasionally. Remove from the heat.

Place a handful of lettuce on a serving plate and spoon the previously made cheese mixture. Top with mushrooms and serve.

Nutrition information per serving: Kcal: 298, Protein: 12.1g, Carbs: 11.9g, Fats: 24.6g

42.   Tuna Stuffed Eggplant

Ingredients:

1 lb of tuna steaks, skinless and boneless

2 medium-sized eggplants, halved

3 tbsp of caper, drained

1 tbsp of olive oil

½ tbsp of butter, melted

2 tbsp of fresh basil, finely chopped

¼ tsp of salt

Preparation:

Preheat the oven to 370°F.

Combine tuna, butter, and capers in a food processor. Blend until smooth and transfer to a medium bowl. Stir in the basil and set aside.

Take a large baking sheet and place some baking paper. Spread the eggplant halves onto it and sprinkle with some olive oil. Put it in the oven and bake until eggplants are fork-tender. Remove from the heat and let it cool for 10 minutes.

Spoon the tuna mixture into each eggplant. Sprinkle with salt to taste. Top with extra capers or grated cheese. Serve.

Nutrition information per serving: Kcal: 322, Protein: 36.1g, Carbs: 16.3g, Fats: 12.6g

43.   Sour Boiled Eggs

Ingredients:

2 medium onions

4 boiled eggs

1 cup of chopped pickles

1 tsp of grated fresh ginger

1 tbsp of low fat cream

1 tbsp of lemon juice

1 tbsp of olive oil

1 tsp of ground turmeric

Salt to taste

Preparation:

Peel and cut the onions. Salt it and leave it to stand for about 5 minutes. Wash and squeeze, and sprinkle some lemon juice over it and leave it.

Add the eggs to a pot of boiling water. Be very gentle while doing this to prevent the eggs to crack.

One useful tip to prepare the perfect eggs is to add 1 tbsp

of baking soda into the boiling water. This will make a peeling process much easier.

Boil the eggs for 8 minutes. You can use a kitchen timer, or simply your watch. After 8 minutes, drain the water and place the eggs under the cold water for few minutes. Peel and slice the eggs.

Combine it with chopped pickles and ginger. Add onions and season with olive oil, low fat cream, salt and turmeric. Serve cold.

Nutrition information per serving: Kcal: 247, Protein: 12.8g, Carbs: 14.2g, Fats: 16.2g

44.   Kiwi Banana Smoothie

Ingredients:

2 medium-sized kiwi, peeled

1 large banana, sliced

1 tbsp of lemon juice

½ cup of Greek yogurt

1 tbsp of honey

Preparation:

Combine all ingredients in a food processor. Blend until smooth. Add few ice cubes and re-blend for 30 seconds. Transfer the mixture to a serving glass. Top with extra honey for sweetness.

Nutrition information per serving: Kcal: 178, Protein: 6.7g, Carbs: 37.5g, Fats: 1.7g

45.   Shrimps in Tomato Sauce with Potatoes

Ingredients:

12 oz of shrimps, peeled and deveined

4 small potatoes, peeled and halved

2 tbsp of heavy cream

4 tbsp of Parmesan cheese, grated

1 tsp of oregano

2 tbsp of olive oil

2 medium-sized tomatoes, blended

¼ tsp of salt

¼ tsp of black pepper, ground

Preparation:

Place potatoes in a large pot over a medium-high temperature. Sprinkle with salt to taste and cook until fork-tender. Remove from the heat and drain. Set aside.

Meanwhile, place tomatoes in blender and blend until smooth. Set aside.

Preheat the oil in a large nonstick skillet over a medium-high temperature. Add shrimps and tomato mixture. Stir well and cook for about 5-6 minutes or until set. Add heavy cream and cheese and give it a good stir. Cook until cheese melts. Remove from the heat and let it cool for a while.

Place potatoes into a serving plate. Spoon the shrimp sauce on top. Sprinkle with oregano to taste and serve.

Nutrition information per serving: Kcal: 317, Protein: 23.1g, Carbs: 30.8g, Fats: 11.6g

46.   Cucumber Quinoa Berry Salad

Ingredients:

1 large cucumber, sliced

1 cup of white quinoa, pre-cooked

1 cup of fresh cranberries

1 cup of fresh blueberries

2 tbsp of almonds, roughly chopped

1 small red onion, diced

1 tsp of maple syrup

1 tbsp of olive oil

2 tbsp of balsamic vinegar

Preparation:

Place quinoa in a large pot. Pour enough water to cover it. Bring it to a boil and then reduce the temperature to low. Cook for about 13-15 minutes and remove from the heat. Fluff with spoon and transfer to a large bowl. Set aside to cool for a while.

Meanwhile, combine oil, vinegar, and maple syrup. Whisk well to combine and pour it over the quinoa.

Now, add cucumbers, onion and fruits and give it a good stir. Set aside or refrigerate for 20 minutes before serving.

Nutrition information per serving: Kcal: 171, Protein: 4.7g, Carbs: 30.4g, Fats: 4.3g

47.   Mixed Berries Pancakes

Ingredients:

3 eggs

½ cup coconut flour

½ cup almond flour

1 cup of coconut milk

1 tsp of apple vinegar

1 tsp vanilla, minced

½ tsp of baking soda

¼ tsp salt

Coconut oil for frying

3 cups of mixed fresh berries

Preparation:

In a large bowl, combine the coconut flour, almond flour, minced vanilla, baking soda, and salt. In a smaller bowl, mix coconut milk and apple vinegar. Whisk in the coconut mixture until smooth dough.

Using a nonstick skillet, heat up the coconut oil over a

medium heat. Spread the desired amount of dough over the skillet. Use a spoon to smooth the surface of each pancake. Fry for about 2-3 minutes on each side.

Top with mixed fresh berries and 1 tbsp of agave syrup.

Nutrition information per serving: Kcal: 186, Protein: 11.9g, Carbs: 55g, Fats: 19.5g

48.   Banana Raisins Cookies

Ingredients:

1 large banana, sliced

¼ cup of dried raisins

1 ½ cup of all-purpose flour

½ tsp of baking powder

1 cup of rolled oats

1 tsp of baking soda

2 tbsp of butter

1 large egg

3 tbsp of honey

1 tsp of vanilla extract

½ cup of dark chocolate, finely chopped

2 tbsp of walnuts, roughly chopped

¼ tsp of salt

Preparation:

Preheat the oven to 375°F.

Combine flour, baking soda, and baking powder in a large bowl. Mix well with a spoon and add honey, butter, salt, banana, and vanilla. Use a hand mixer to combine and mix until you get thick batter. Form the cookies with hands and roll into the rolled oats, chocolate chops, raisins, and walnuts.

Line some parchment paper over a baking sheet and spread the cookies. Make 1 inch space between the cookies. Put it in the oven and bake for about 10-15 minutes or until golden brown and crisp. Remove from the heat and set aside to cool before serving.

Nutrition information per serving: Kcal: 562, Protein: 10.3g, Carbs: 90.2g, Fats: 17.5g

49.   Rice Pilaf with Spinach

Ingredients:

1 cup of brown rice, pre-cooked, drained and rinsed

1 lb of fresh spinach, pre-cooked

1 garlic clove, minced

1 small onion, diced

1 tbsp of vegetable oil

1 tsp of dried thyme, ground

¼ cup of cheddar cheese, shredded

2 large eggs

Preparation:

Preheat the oven to 350°F.

Place rice in a large pot and pour water enough to cover it. Cook for 30 minutes or until almost done. Remove from the heat. Drain and rinse few times with cold water. Set aside.

Place spinach in the same pot and pour enough water to cover it. Cook until soften. Remove from the heat and set aside.

Preheat the oil in the same pot and add onion and garlic. Stir-fry until translucent and remove from the heat.

Now, combine pre-cooked rice and spinach, cheese, and thyme in a large mixing bowl. Beat the egg Into the bowl and give it a good stir to combine. Sprinkle a pinch of salt to taste and set aside.

Grease a nonstick baking sheet and spread the mixture evenly. Cover with aluminum foil and put it in the oven. Bake for about 20-25 minutes. Remove the foil, and bake for another 5-6 minutes. Remove from the heat and make 4 equal portions.

You can top with one tablespoon of sour cream. However, this is optional.

Nutrition information per serving: Kcal: 301, Protein: 12.2g, Carbs: 42.3g, Fats: 10.3g

50. Trout with Veggies

Ingredients:

2 lbs of trout fillet, boneless

1 medium-sized tomato, wedged

1 medium-sized bell pepper, cut into strips

1 small onion, sliced

3 tbsp of lemon juice

3 tbsp of cilantro, chopped

1 tsp of rosemary, finely chopped

¼ tsp of sea salt

¼ tsp of black pepper, ground

Preparation:

Preheat oven to 350 °F.

Wash, pat dry, and place the filets in a large greased baking dish.

Combine tomato, pepper, onion, lemon juice, cilantro, salt, and pepper in a mixing bowl. Stir well and spoon the mixture over the fillets. Place it in the oven and bake for

20 minutes, or until fish fork-tender.

Nutrition information per serving: Kcal: 305, Protein: 34.2g, Carbs: 4.3, Fats: 11.4g

51.   Potato Salad

Ingredients:

3 lbs large potatoes, pre-cooked

1 cup of fresh celery, chopped

½ cup of spring onions, chopped

¼ cup of sour cream

½ cup of cottage cheese, crumbled

1 tbsp of lemon juice

1 tsp of apple cider vinegar

½ tbsp of yellow mustard

¼ tsp of salt

¼ tsp of black pepper, ground

Preparation:

Place potatoes in a pot of boiling water and cook until fork-tender. Drain and set aside to cool.

Combine potatoes, spring onions, celery, parsley, and green onions in a large bowl. Set aside.

Meanwhile, combine sour cream, lemon juice, vinegar,

mustard, salt, and pepper in a food processor. Blend until smooth and pour over the previously prepared salad. Refrigerate for 1 hour before serving.

Nutrition information per serving: Kcal: 302, Protein: 9.8g, Carbs: 57.1, Fats: 4.2g

ADDITIONAL TITLES FROM THIS AUTHOR

70 Effective Meal Recipes to Prevent and Solve Being Overweight: Burn Fat Fast by Using Proper Dieting and Smart Nutrition

By

Joe Correa CSN

48 Acne Solving Meal Recipes: The Fast and Natural Path to Fixing Your Acne Problems in Less Than 10 Days!

By

Joe Correa CSN

41 Alzheimer's Preventing Meal Recipes: Reduce or Eliminate Your Alzheimer's Condition in 30 Days or Less!

By

Joe Correa CSN

70 Effective Breast Cancer Meal Recipes: Prevent and Fight Breast Cancer with Smart Nutrition and Powerful Foods

By

Joe Correa CSN